Copyright © 2020 by Verona Jackson

RND

All rights reserved. No part of this publication may be reproduced, distributed, or transmitted in any form or by any means, including photocopying, recording, or other electronic or mechanical methods, without the prior written permission of the publisher, except in the case of brief quotations embodied in critical reviews and certain other noncommercial uses permitted by copyright law

Table of Contents

Table of Contents 2

Introduction 5

Gluten-Free Snacks Recipes for You 7

   Crackers Snack 7

   Hardboiled Eggs 8

   Dried Apricots & Almonds 10

   Tropical Yogurt Parfait 10

   Peanut Butter & Apple Slices 12

   PB Granola Bars 13

   Peanuts & Raisins 15

   Power Smoothie 16

Peanut Butter & Banana 17

Nachos 18

Popcorn & String Cheese 20

Trail Mix 20

Stuffed Quesadilla 21

Dark Chocolate Covered Almonds 24

S'Mores 25

Coconut Chia Pudding 26

Cookie Truffles 27

Lowfat Vanilla/Strawberry Ice Cream 29

Popcorn Balls 30

Peanut Butter Cookies 32

Funky Feta Skewers 33

Salmon & Lemon Mini Fish Cakes 35

Parmesan, Poppy Seed & Caraway Twists 38

Sesame & Chilli Pancakes with Tzatziki 41

Spiced Sweet Potato Wedges 43

Gluten-Free Hot Cross Buns 45

Gluten-Free Lemon Drizzle Cake 50

Dried Fruit Energy Nuggets 52

Chinese-Spiced Seed Mix 54

Halloumi & Bacon Rolls 55

Glamorgan Cheese Sausage Rolls 57

Mini Jacket Potatoes 60

Courgette & Halloumi Skewers 62

Introduction

Humans generally expecially kids typically love to munch on different treats, and eating healthy snacks throughout the day can boost your energy and nutritional intake. Keeping your yourselves or kids gluten-free, though, can be challenging, especially when it comes to snacks. By the time you finally find the right afternoon fix, you or your kid is likely already in the middle of a meltdown. Lucky for you, help is on the way with these easy and gluten-free snacks.

Gluten is a protein found in wheat, barley, rye, and triticale. If you or your child has celiac disease or a gluten intolerance, you already know that they should avoid all products made with gluten-containing grains. For them, eating gluten could result in serious side effects such as: anemia, malnutrition, rash or eczema, joint pain, headaches, fatigue or nervous system issues

So, arm yourself with the right ingredients and a little knowledge, and you'll keep yourself or kids gluten-free and healthy.

Gluten-Free Snacks Recipes for You

Crackers Snack

Ingredients

- Milton's Gluten-Free Crackers
- cream cheese
- Dill
- Cracked Black Pepper

or

- Milton's Gluten-Free Crackers
- Bacon Bits
- Egg sliced thinly

Instructions

1. Smear cream cheese on crackers and sprinkle with dill and freshly cracked black pepper.

or

2. Top crackers with a small slice of bacon and a sliver of boiled egg.

Hardboiled Eggs

Ingredients

- 1 dozen Eggs

- 1 dash Salt

Instructions

3. Place one dozen eggs in a large pot of tap-temperature water and add a dash of salt.
4. Turn heat to medium and bring water and eggs to a boil.
5. Once at a boil, remove the pot from the heat and cover with lid for 12 minutes.
6. Rinse eggs under cool water to prevent the "green ring" from forming around the yolk.

Dried Apricots & Almonds

Ingredients

- 1 Handfull Dried Apricots
- 1 Handfull Almonds

Instructions

1. Mix ingredeints together & enjoy!

Tropical Yogurt Parfait

Ingredients

- 1 Pint So Delicious Dairy Free Vanilla Yogurt or plain yogurt

- 1 Cup Gluten-Free Graham Crackers crushed
- 1 Sliced Star Fruit
- 1/2 Cup Tropical Fruit diced
- 1/2 Cup Mixed Berries
- 1/4 Cup Coconut toasted, shredded
- 4 Martini or Margarita Glasses

Instructions

2. Spoon dollop of yogurt into base of martini or other festive glass; top with sprinkling of gluten-free graham crackers, followed by layer of diced fruit and a few berries.
3. Repeat pattern until glass is filled, placing star fruit slices in center on top.

4. Sprinkle with 1/4 of toasted coconut.

5. Assemble remaining 3 parfaits.

Peanut Butter & Apple Slices

Ingredients

- 1 Medium Apple
- 2-4 Tablespoons Peanut Butter

Instructions

1. Core and slice apple into wedges.

2. Divide the peanut butter evenly among the slices. Enjoy!

PB Granola Bars

Ingredients

- 1/3 cup honey
- 1/4 cup Peanut Butter natural
- 2 tbsp Butter unsalted
- 1 cup rice cereal crisp

- 1 cup gluten free rolled oats
- 1/4 cup Dried Fruit
- 2 scoops protein powder optional
- 2 tbsp flaxseed ground, optional

Instructions

1. In a saucepan over heat, add honey, peanut butter, and butter. Stir until loosened and smooth (about 1-2 minutes).
2. Remove from heat.
3. Stir in cereal, oats, dried fruit, and other optional ingredients.

4. Drop a tablespoonful of mixture into each lined cupcake tin, or spread in baking tin approximately 1/2 inch thick.

5. Refrigerate approximately 15 minutes until set.

6. For bars, cut with sharp knife and remove from pan with spatula.

Peanuts & Raisins

Ingredients

- 1 Handfull Peanuts
- 1 Handfull Raisins

Instructions

1. Mix ingredeints together & enjoy!

Power Smoothie

Ingredients

- 2 Cups Spinach fresh
- 1 Tablespoon Hodgson Mill Ground Flaxseed
- 1/2 Cup Almond Milk
- 1 Cup berries frozen
- Banana
- 1 Tablespoon Nut Butter

Instructions

1. Blend ingredients and serve!

Peanut Butter & Banana

Ingredients

- 1 Medium Banana
- Tablespoons Peanut Butter

Instructions

2. Slice bananas into 1/2 thick slices and lay out on a cookie sheet.

3 Spread an even amount of peanut butter over top of the slices and enjoy!

Nachos

Ingredients

- 8 Ounces Mission Gluten-Free Tortilla Chips
- 1 Can Refried Beans
- 1/2 Cup Sour Cream
- 8 Ounces Shredded Mexican Cheese Blend
- 1 Cup Roma Tomato diced

Instructions

1. Preheat your oven to 375 degrees. Line 2 large baking sheets with foil or parchment paper.
2. Place the chips in a single layer on the prepared pans.
3. Spread the beans on the chips, dividing evenly between the two pans.
4. Sprinkle the pans with the cheese. Place the baking sheets in the oven and bake for 5 minutes, or until the cheese is melted.
5. Serve & Enjoy!

Popcorn & String Cheese

Ingredients

- 1 Handfull Popcorn
- 1 Stick String Cheese

Instructions

1. Place together in a plate and enjoy!

Trail Mix

Ingredients

- 1/2 Cup Cashews

- 1/4 Cup Peanuts
- 1/4 Cup Almonds
- 1/2 Cup Raisins
- 1/4 Cup Enjoy Life Chocolate Chips

Instructions

1. Mix ingredients together and enjoy!

Stuffed Quesadilla

Ingredients

- 2 Udi's Gluten-Free Large Tortillas

- 1 Cup Cheddar Cheese shredded
- 1/4 Cup chicken grilled, skinless, cubed
- 1/4 Cup Potatoes peeled, precooked, cubed
- 1/4 Cup Bell Pepper roasted, cubed
- 1/4 Cup Black Beans cooked and strained
- 1/4 Cup Artichoke Hearts chopped
- 1/4 Cup Corn kernels, cooked
- 1/4 Cup Carrots shredded

Instructions

2. Preheat a griddle or nonstick pan over medium heat.

3. Place the first tortilla on the griddle and flip it over when it starts to smoke.

4. Top with 1/2 cup cheese and sprinkle the chicken over the cheese.
5. Spread potatoes over chicken and top with peppers and black beans.
6. Add artichoke hearts, corn, and carrots.
7. Add the remaining 1/2 cup cheese and top with the second tortilla.
8. Cook about 10 minutes, until the cheese is melted.
9. Flip the quesadilla and cook another five minutes.
10. Remove from the pan.
11. Cut in fourths and serve with salsa or sour cream.

Dark Chocolate Covered Almonds

Ingredients

- 8 Ounces Enjoy Life Dark Chocolate
- 2 Cups Unsalted Raw Almonds

Instructions

1. Melt the chocolate in a double boiler over medium heat. Stir until melted.
2. Stir the almonds into the chocolate, and toss until well coated.
3. Place the chocolate covered almonds onto a parchment paper covered baking sheet.
4. Store in the refrigerator until ready to eat.

S'Mores

Ingredients

- 1 Large Marshmallow
- 1 Pamela's Products Graham Cracker
- 1 Ounce Chocolate

Instructions

1. Heat the marshmallow over flame until it begins to brown. Break the graham cracker in half.
2. Sandwich the chocolate between the cracker and the hot marshmallow.
3. Allow the marshmallow to cool before eating.

Coconut Chia Pudding

Ingredients

Pudding

- 1/4 Cup Coco Libre Coconut Water
- 1 Cup Coconut Milk
- 2 Tablespoons Chia Seeds
- 1 Teaspoon Vanilla Extract

Toppings

- 1/2 Cup Fresh Fruit blueberries, strawberries, kiwi, raspberries etc.
- 1/4 Cup Raw Nuts chopped
- 2 Teaspoons honey optional

Instructions

1. Combine pudding ingredients and whisk until well blended.

2. Cover and let sit for a few hours or overnight.

3. Just before serving, add fruits, nuts, and honey.

Cookie Truffles

Ingredients

- 10 Dates pitted

- NoGii Protein D'Lites Chocolate Caramel Bliss Bars
- 1/4 Cup powdered sugar
- 1/8 Teaspoon Sea Salt
- 1/2 Teaspoon Vanilla Extract

Instructions

1. Place the dates in a small bowl and cover with hot water to soak for 10–20 minutes, or until softened.
2. Once softened, combine in a food processor with the Protein D'Lites Chocolate Caramel Bliss bars, vanilla extract, and sea salt.

3   Pulse the machine until the mixture is roughly combined.

4   Scoop out 1/2–1 tablespoon of the dough at a time and roll into small balls with your hands.

5   Roll the balls in the powdered sugar, and set aside in the refrigerator to chill for 10 minutes.

Lowfat Vanilla/Strawberry Ice Cream

Ingredients

- Vanilla ice cream

- Strawberry ice cream

Instructions

1. Scoop, and enjoy!

Popcorn Balls

Ingredients

- tbsp Butter
- 1 bag marshmallows mini
- 12 cups Popcorn plain, unsalted, popped

- 1/2 cup Cashews unsalted
- 1/2 cup Raisins

Instructions

2   Melt butter in saucepan over low heat.

3   Add marshmallows and stir until melted, approximately 10-12 minutes.

4   Pour out unpopped kernels from popcorn.

5   In a large bowl, combine popcorn, cashews, and raisins.

6   Pour melted marshmallows over popcorn mixture and fold to combine.

7   Rub hands with butter to prevent sticking. Form 12 balls approximately 2 1/2 inches

wide and place on wax paper to cool (about 10 minutes).

Peanut Butter Cookies

Ingredients

- 1 Cup Peanut Butter
- 1 Cup Sugar
- 2 Eggs
- 1 Teaspoon Bob's Red Mill Double Acting Baking Powder
- 1 Teaspoon Bob's Red Mill Pure Baking Soda

Instructions

1 Preheat oven to 350°F.

2 Combine all ingredients in a large bowl until blended.

3 Roll dough into tablespoon-sized balls.

4 Bake 12-15 minutes.

Funky Feta Skewers

Ingredients

- 1 large mango, peeled and chunkily diced into 10

- about 300g watermelon
- flesh, diced into 10
- 200g pack feta cheese, cut into 20 cubes
- 1 tsp poppy seed, toasted
- 20 mini skewers, to serve
- 1 citrus fruit, to serve (optional)
- 1 lime

Instructions

1. Put the mango on one plate, melon on another and feta on a third.
2. Scatter some poppy seeds over each, and gently toss so the seeds stick.

3   Assemble 10 skewers with cubes of mango and feta, and 10 skewers with cubes of melon and feta.

4   Stick into citrus fruit, if you like, or arrange on a platter, and squeeze over the lime. Cover and chill until about 20 mins before serving.

Salmon & Lemon Mini Fish Cakes

Ingredients

- 2 large baking potatoes
- 2 tbsp olive oil

- grated zest and juice ½ lemon
- 1 egg yolk
- 140g smoked salmon trimmings, plus extra to serve
- 1 tbsp chopped parsley, plust extra
- 2 tbsp gluten-free flour mixed with 1 tsp coarsely ground pepper
- a little oil, for frying

Instructions

1. Microwave potatoes on high for 10 mins until tender. Leave to cool for 5 mins, scoop the flesh in a bowl, then mash and leave to cool.

2. Season with olive oil, lemon zest and juice to taste, then mix in the egg, salmon and parsley.

3. Shape into small rounds 3cm wide and 1cm deep. Chill for 15 mins.

4. Dust each cake with the peppered flour, then fry over a low heat in a little oil for 2-3 mins on each side.

5. Drain on kitchen paper and serve garnished with salmon and parsley.

Parmesan, Poppy Seed & Caraway Twists

Ingredients

- 175g gluten-free flour
- 85g butter
- pinch cayenne pepper
- 1 egg yolk mixed with 3 tbsp cold water
- 1 egg, beaten
- tbsp freshly grated parmesan (or vegetarian alternative)
- 1 tbsp each poppy seeds and caraway seeds

Instructions

1 To make the pastry, put the flour, butter and cayenne pepper into a food processor, then whizz into fine breadcrumbs.

2 sprinkle the egg and water mixture onto the flour, then pulse again until the mixture begins to come together.

3 Tip the mixture onto a board and gently squeeze the pastry until it begins to come together in a ball, adding more water if it feels dry.

4 Heat oven to 190C/fan 170C/gas 5. roll the pastry into a large a4-sized rectangle, roughly 20 x 30cm.

5 Brush the sheet with the beaten egg and cut in half widthways.

6 Sprinkle one half with the Parmesan and the second half with poppy and caraway seeds.

7 lightly run the rolling pin across the top to press the cheese and the seeds into the pastry.

8 Cut each half into 12-15 sticks. arrange on a baking sheet and chill for 10 mins.

9 Bake for 8-10 mins until golden brown, then cool for 5 mins before lifting onto a wire rack.

Sesame & Chilli Pancakes with Tzatziki

Ingredients

- 100g gluten-free flour
- 1 egg
- 150ml soya yogurt
- 1 green and 1 red chilli, deseeded and finely chopped
- 1 bunch spring onions, finely sliced, plus extra to serve
- 2 tbsp chopped coriander
- 1 tbsp sesame seeds
- a little oil for frying
- For the tzatziki
- 150g Greek yogurt
- 13cm/5in cucumber, deseeded and grated

- 2 tbsp chopped mint

Instructions

1 Whizz the flour, egg, yogurt and 2 tbsp water together in a food processor to form a smooth batter.

2 Tip into a bowl, then stir in the chillies, spring onions, coriander and sesame seeds. Cover and chill until required.

3 To make the tzatziki, mix the yogurt, cucumber and mint together, season to taste, then chill.

4 Heat a small frying pan with a splash of oil, wiping out excess oil with kitchen paper.

5 Fry the pancake mixture a dessertspoonful at a time, for 1 min on each side, until lightly browned.

6 Tip onto a plate and keep warm. pile onto a large platter, top with a dollop of tzatziki and some extra sliced spring onions and serve warm.

Spiced Sweet Potato Wedges

Ingredients

- 2 tsp ground cumin
- 2 tsp chilli flakes

- 2 tsp sumac
- 2 tbsp thyme leaves, roughly chopped
- 2 tbsp rosemary leaves, roughly chopped
- garlic cloves
- zest and juice 1 lemon
- 3 tbsp olive oil
- 1¼kg sweet potatoes, cut into wedges

Instructions

1. Heat oven to 200C/180C fan/gas 6.
2. Using a pestle and mortar, bash together the spices, herbs, garlic and some seasoning.
3. Spoon into a large bowl and stir in the lemon zest and juice, and the oil.

4 Add the potatoes and toss together.

5 Arrange, skin-side down, on 2 baking trays and bake for 30–40 mins until soft inside and crisp on the outside.

Gluten-Free Hot Cross Buns

Ingredients

- 300ml full-fat milk, plus 2 tbsp more
- 50g butter
- 500g gluten and wheat-free white bread

- 1 tsp salt
- 75g caster sugar
- 1 tbsp sunflower oil
- 2 tsp quick or fast-action yeast
- 1 large egg, beaten
- 1 tsp olive oil
- 75g sultana
- 50g mixed peel
- zest 1 orange
- 1 apple, peeled, cored and finely chopped
- 1 tsp ground cinnamon

For the cross

- 30g gluten and wheat-free plain flour, plus extra for dusting

For the glaze

- tbsp apricot jam

Instructions

1 Bring the milk to the boil, then remove from the heat and add the butter. Leave to cool until it reaches hand temperature.

2 Mix the flour, salt, sugar and yeast with the warm milk and egg in a mixer with a dough attachment, or with a wooden spoon.

3 Then bring together the dough with your hands. Don't knead.

4 Put the dough in a lightly oiled bowl. Cover with oiled cling film and leave to rise in a

warm place for 1 hr or until doubled in size and a finger pressed into it leaves a dent.

5 Tip in the olive oil, sultanas, mixed peel, orange zest, apple and cinnamon and mix into the dough.

6 Shape into buns by lightly oiling your hands and dividing the dough into 100g pieces before rolling into balls. Leave to rise for another hour.

7 Heat oven to 220C/200C fan/gas 7.

8 Mix the flour with about 3 tbsp water to make the paste for the cross

9 Add the water 1 tbsp at a time, so you add just enough for a thick paste. Spoon into a piping bag with a small nozzle.

10 Pipe a line along each row of buns, then repeat in the other direction to create crosses.

11 Bake for 20 mins on the middle shelf of the oven, until golden brown.

12 Gently heat the apricot jam to melt, then sieve to get rid of any chunks.

13 While the jam is still warm, brush over the top of the warm buns and serve.

Gluten-Free Lemon Drizzle Cake

Ingredients

- 200g butter, softened
- 200g golden caster sugar
- eggs
- 175g ground almond (switch for polenta or wheat-free flour to make this recipe nut-free)
- 250g mashed potato
- zest 3 lemons
- 2 tsp gluten-free baking powder

For the drizzle

- tbsp granulated sugar
- juice 1 lemon

Instructions

1 Heat oven to 180C/fan 160C/gas 4. Butter and line a deep, 20cm round cake tin.

2 Beat the sugar and butter together until light and fluffy, then gradually add the egg, beating after each addition.

3 Fold in the almonds, cold mashed potato, lemon zest and baking powder.

4 Tip into the tin, level the top, then bake for 40-45 mins or until golden and a skewer inserted into the middle of the cake comes out clean.

5 Turn out onto a wire rack after 10 mins cooling. Mix the granulated sugar and the lemon juice together.

6   Then spoon over the top of the cake, letting it drip down the sides. Let the cake cool completely before slicing.

Dried Fruit Energy Nuggets

Ingredients

- 50g soft dried apricot
- 100g soft dried date
- 50g dried cherry

- 2 tsp coconut oil
- 1 tbsp toasted sesame seed

Instructions

1. Whizz apricots with dates and cherries in a food processor until very finely chopped.
2. Tip into a bowl and use your hands to work in coconut oil.
3. Shape the mix into walnut-sized balls, then roll in sesame seeds.
4. Store in an airtight container until you need a quick energy fix.

Chinese-Spiced Seed Mix

Ingredients

- 1 egg white
- 2 tsp Chinese five-spice powder
- ½ tsp salt
- 85g each sunflower and pumpkin seed

Instructions

1. Heat oven to 150C/130C fan/gas 2. Lightly whisk egg white, then add Chinese five spice and salt.
2. Add sunflower and pumpkin seeds, and coat well. Spread out in a single layer on a lightly oiled baking sheet and bake for 12 mins.

3   Cool before eating.

Halloumi & Bacon Rolls

Ingredients

- 250g block halloumi cheese
- rashers pancetta or smoked streaky bacon
- 1 tbsp chopped chives

Instructions

1. Heat oven to 200C/fan 180C/gas 6. Cut the halloumi into 20 sticks.
2. Stretch each rasher of pancetta with the back of a knife, then cut in half.
3. Season the pancetta with just black pepper, then sprinkle with the chopped chives.
4. Roll the pancetta around the halloumi in a spiral and arrange on a baking sheet.
5. Bake for 10-12 mins or until the pancetta is brown and beginning to crisp.

Glamorgan Cheese Sausage Rolls

Ingredients

For the pastry

- 175g gluten-free flour
- 85g butter
- pinch cayenne pepper
- 1 egg yolk mixed with 3 tbsp cold water
- For the filling
- 100g gluten-free breadcrumbs
- 100g Caerphilly cheese, grated
- 1 small leek, finely chopped
- 1 tsp mustard seeds, crushed
- egg yolks

- handful tarragon or thyme leaves **(optional)**

Instructions

1 To make the pastry, put the flour, butter and cayenne pepper into a food processor, then whizz into fine breadcrumbs.

2 Sprinkle the egg and water mixture onto the flour and pulse again until the mixture begins to come together.

3 Tip the mixture onto a board, then gently squeeze the pastry until it begins to come together in a ball, adding more water if it feels dry.

4 Divide the mixture in half, roll each piece into a 12 x 30cm rectangle and slip onto a baking sheet. Do not chill.

5 Heat oven to 200C/fan 180C/gas 6. Mix the filling ingredients together, except one egg yolk, which you need for glazing, in a food processor.

6 Divide in two and roll each into a 30cm-long sausage shape. Lay a cheese sausage on one side of the pastry.

7 Brush the sausage and pastry with egg yolk and fold the pastry over the top to encase the sausage.

8. Seal the two edges, trim the ends, then cut into 2cm pieces. Arrange on a baking sheet and chill for 30 mins.

9. Brush the rolls with a little more egg yolk, place herbs on top, if you like

10. Then bake for 12-15 mins until golden brown.

Mini Jacket Potatoes

Ingredients

- 500g bag new potato
- 1 tbsp olive oil

- sea salt
- 75ml half-fat soured cream
- small bunch chives, snipped

Instructions

1 Heat oven to 190C/170C fan/gas 5. Prick the potatoes with a fork, rub with the oil, then toss with sea salt.

2 Arrange on a baking sheet and bake for 1 hr.

3 Let the potatoes cool for 10-15 mins, then cut a small cross in the top of each and pinch the bases to open a little.

4   Add a teaspoon of soured cream to each, a little freshly ground black pepper, and a sprinkling of chives.

5   Serve straightway.

Courgette & Halloumi Skewers

Ingredients

- ½ tsp chilli powder
- small handful mint, chopped
- zest and juice 1 lemon

- 2 tbsp extra-virgin olive oil
- 2 courgettes, cut into 1cm rounds
- 225g pack halloumi cheese, cubed

Instructions

1. Mix the chilli, half the mint, lemon zest and juice, oil, courgettes and halloumi.
2. Leave to marinate for 30 mins. Soak 8 wooden skewers for 20 mins.
3. Thread the courgettes and halloumi onto the skewers. Cook on the BBQ, or under a grill, for 7-8 mins, turning halfway through and basting with the remaining marinade. Scatter over remaining mint.

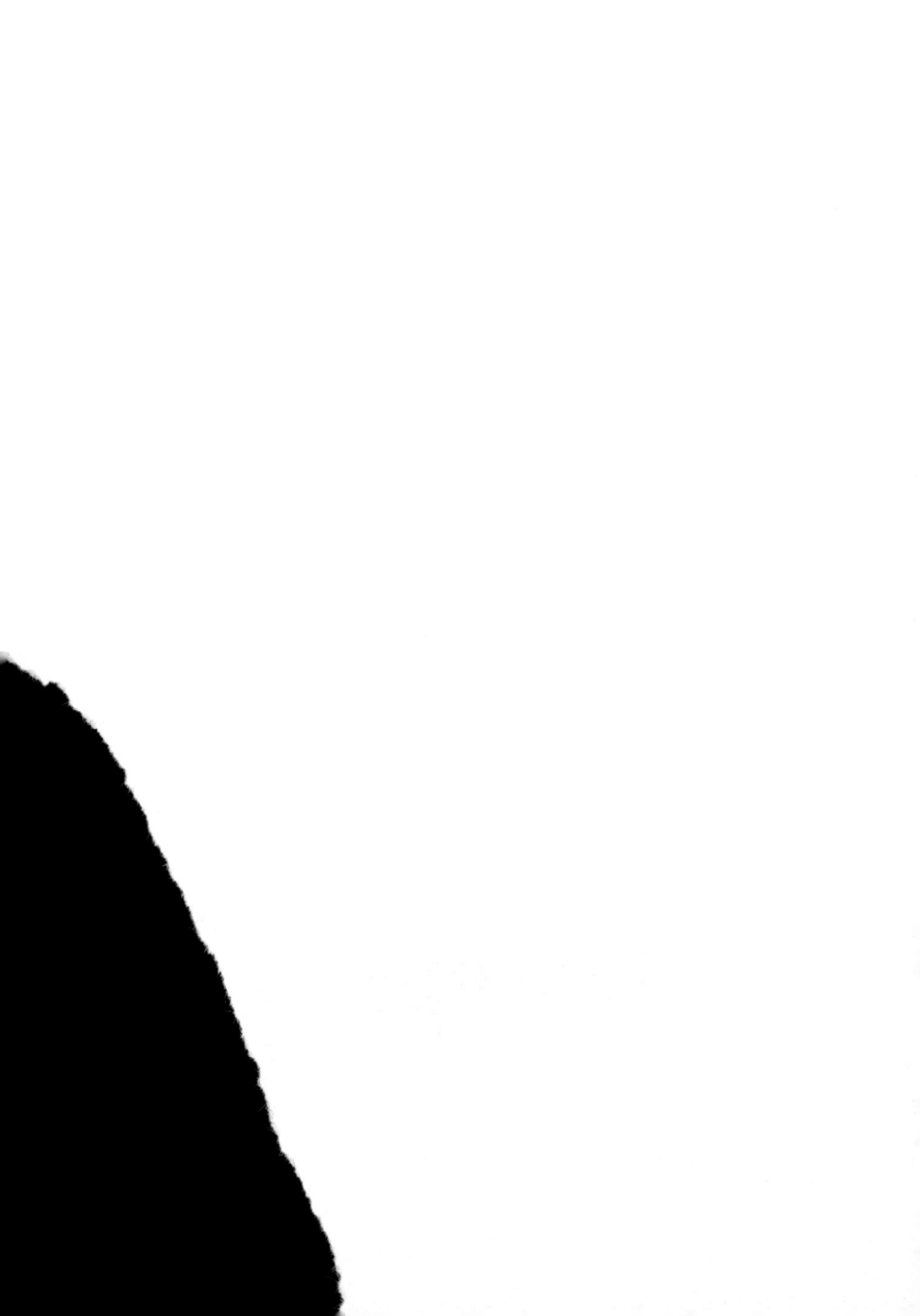

Made in the USA
Las Vegas, NV
21 August 2023